The Doctor's Conscience

Navigating Patient Autonomy and Physician Responsibility in Modern Healthcare

Essie Hunter

Table of Contents

1 **Chapter 1: The Ethical Framework** **5**
1.1 Autonomy's Cornerstone 7
1.2 Beneficence & Non-Maleficence 9
1.3 Justice in Healthcare 12

2 **Chapter 2: Informed Consent** **15**
2.1 Legal Aspects 17
2.2 Practical Application 19

3 **Chapter 3: End-of-Life Care** **23**
3.1 Advanced Directives 25
3.2 Palliative Care 27
3.3 Withdrawing Treatment 29
3.4 Physician-Assisted Suicide 31
3.5 Euthanasia 33

4 **Chapter 4: Resource Allocation** **37**
4.1 Scarcity & Prioritization 39
4.2 Ethical Dilemmas 41

5 **Chapter 5: Medical Error & Disclosure** **45**
5.1 Transparency & Trust 47
5.2 Legal Ramifications 49
5.3 Patient Communication 53

6 Chapter 6: Confidentiality & Privacy **57**
6.1 HIPAA & Beyond 59
6.2 Exceptions to Confidentiality 61

7 Chapter 7: The Future of Ethics **65**
7.1 Technological Advancements 67
7.2 Global Healthcare 69
7.3 Maintaining Integrity 71
7.4 Emerging Challenges 73
7.5 Professional Responsibility 76

1 Chapter 1: The Ethical Framework

Respect for patient autonomy forms the bedrock of ethical medical practice. It's not merely about obtaining consent; it's about empowering individuals to make informed decisions concerning their own bodies and health, acknowledging their unique values and preferences. This requires physicians to actively foster open communication, patiently explaining medical complexities in a way patients can readily understand. Failure to do so undermines this fundamental right, potentially leading to resentment, distrust, and ultimately, suboptimal care. A physician's role transcends technical expertise; it demands empathy, active listening, and a genuine commitment to supporting the patient's self-determination, even when it differs from our own clinical judgment. True patient-centered care necessitates this unwavering respect for autonomy.

Beneficence, the commitment to act in the patient's best interest, is intrinsically linked to non-maleficence, the duty to avoid causing harm. These principles, though seemingly straightforward, often present complex challenges in practice. For example, a treatment offering potential benefit might also carry significant risks. The physician's ethical responsibility lies in carefully weighing these factors, fully informing the patient, and collaboratively deciding on a course of action that aligns with the patient's values and minimizes potential harm. This delicate balancing act requires sound clinical judgment, a deep understanding of the patient's individual circumstances, and an unwavering commitment to acting in their best interests. It's not about imposing our own view of "best" but rather a shared decision-making process guided by ethical principles and sound medical evidence.

Justice in healthcare demands equitable access to quality care, regardless of factors like socioeconomic status, race, ethnicity, or geographic location. This principle underscores the moral obligation to address healthcare disparities and advocate for policies that promote fair resource allocation. We must critically examine systems that perpetuate inequalities, striving to ensure that all individuals have equal opportunities to achieve optimal health outcomes. This requires a societal commitment to healthcare as a fundamental human right and challenges us to address systemic issues that create barriers to access. The pursuit of justice demands not only individual commitment but also collective action to create a fairer and more equitable healthcare system. It requires active engagement in advocacy and policy reform to bring about meaningful change. The physician has a critical role to play, advocating for their patients and contributing towards a just healthcare system that serves all.

Navigating these principles requires ongoing self-reflection and critical analysis. Ethical dilemmas are inevitable, often involving difficult choices with no easy answers. A commitment to continuous ethical learning, seeking guidance from experienced colleagues or ethics committees when needed, and engaging in open dialogue with patients are essential tools. The goal isn't to find perfect solutions but to engage in a thoughtful, deliberate process guided by ethical principles, striving always to act with integrity and compassion. This journey of ethical practice is ongoing, a constant striving to uphold the highest standards of patient care and professional responsibility. We must embrace this challenge, continuously refining our approaches to ensure we remain true to the ethical foundation of medicine.

The application of these principles is not confined to clinical encounters; it extends to all aspects of professional conduct. Maintaining professional boundaries, adhering to high standards of clinical competence, and engaging in honest self-reflection are all integral to ethical medical practice. A physician's actions, both within and outside the clinical setting, reflect on the profession as a whole and contribute to public trust. Transparency, accountability, and a commitment to continuous improvement are vital aspects of upholding the integrity of the medical profession. We are accountable not only to our individual patients but to the wider community and to the standards expected of medical professionals.

Ethical decision-making in medicine often necessitates balancing competing principles. Situations may arise where upholding one principle compromises another. For example, respecting patient autonomy might conflict with the physician's duty to promote beneficence, particularly in cases where the patient's choice might lead to harm. These challenging situations demand careful consideration, thoughtful deliberation, and a willingness to engage in difficult conversations with patients and their families. The physician's role, in these cases, is not to make the decision for the patient, but to provide guidance, support, and facilitate a shared decision-making process that respects the patient's autonomy while acknowledging potential risks and benefits.

The ethical framework outlined here provides a fundamental guide, but its practical application requires constant reflection and adjustment. The context surrounding each clinical decision influences the weight given to each ethical principle. Culture, individual beliefs, and societal norms all impact the interpretation and application of these guiding principles. Understanding this requires cultural sensitivity, adaptability, and a recognition that ethical considerations are not static, but evolve within dynamic contexts. Therefore, ongoing education and engagement with the evolving landscape of medical ethics are crucial for continued ethical practice.

1.1 Autonomy's Cornerstone

Respect for patient autonomy isn't merely a legal requirement; it's the moral bedrock of effective healthcare. It acknowledges the inherent dignity of each individual, recognizing their right to make informed decisions about their own bodies and lives, even when those choices differ from medical recommendations. This respect fosters trust, a crucial element in the therapeutic relationship.

Understanding autonomy extends beyond simply informing patients of treatment options. It demands a deep appreciation of their values, beliefs, and life goals. A patient's preference for a less aggressive treatment, even if statistically less effective, must be honored if it aligns with their personal priorities. The physician's role shifts from solely directing treatment to facilitating informed self-determination.

Consider Mrs. Gable, a 78-year-old woman with a history of heart failure. Her recent diagnosis of advanced lung cancer presents a complex challenge. Aggressive chemotherapy offers a statistically small chance of remission, but it comes with debilitating side effects, significantly impacting her quality of life in her remaining time. Mrs. Gable, prioritizing comfort and time with her family over aggressive treatment, opts for palliative care. Respecting her autonomy means supporting her choice, even if it deviates from a purely medically-driven approach.

However, respecting autonomy doesn't equate to absolute patient control. Physicians retain a critical role in providing clear, unbiased information, facilitating thoughtful deliberation, and ensuring patients understand the potential implications of their choices. This requires effective communication tailored to the individual's level of understanding, employing empathy and active listening. It necessitates addressing anxieties and misconceptions, ensuring that the patient's decision is truly informed, rather than based on misinformation or fear.

Navigating situations where patient autonomy conflicts with other ethical principles, such as beneficence, can present significant challenges. For instance, a patient refusing life-saving treatment presents a moral quandary. While respecting autonomy is paramount, the physician's obligation to do no harm and act in the best interest of the patient remains. In these cases, thoughtful dialogue is essential, exploring underlying reasons for refusal and seeking common ground. Perhaps the patient's fear stems from a misunderstanding of the procedure or a lack of trust. Addressing these concerns may lead to a revised decision, one where both autonomy and beneficence are upheld.

The capacity for autonomy is also crucial. Patients with impaired cognitive function, mental illness, or conditions affecting decision-making capability may require additional considerations. In these cases, legal frameworks and ethical guidelines often stipulate the involvement of surrogate decision-makers, usually family members or legal guardians. However, the focus always remains on the best interests of the patient, interpreted within the broadest possible understanding of their prior wishes and values, documented or expressed through prior conversations. It's a delicate balance.

Documentation plays a vital role in safeguarding patient autonomy. Meticulous records of discussions, the information provided, and the patient's decisions demonstrate that the principle of autonomy has been meticulously followed. These records not only protect the physician from potential legal repercussions but also serve as a testament to the collaborative and respectful nature of the doctor-patient relationship. This clear and comprehensive record is vital if disputes arise later or alternative care pathways are needed.

Maintaining a culture that genuinely values patient autonomy necessitates ongoing education and professional reflection. Healthcare providers must constantly evaluate their practices, seeking feedback to enhance communication skills and improve their understanding of individual patient needs. This continuous self-assessment, complemented by interprofessional dialogues, helps foster a healthcare environment centered on collaboration, respect, and a dedication to ethically sound practice. Only then can we truly fulfill our responsibility to our patients. Autonomy, therefore, is not merely a principle to be applied, but a foundational element of trust, respect, and collaborative care that must be nurtured at every step.

1.2 Beneficence & Non-Maleficence

Beneficence, the act of doing good, and non-maleficence, the avoidance of harm, form the bedrock of medical ethics. These principles, seemingly straightforward, present complex challenges in daily practice. Consider a patient with a life-threatening illness; aggressive treatment offers a chance of survival but carries significant risks, including debilitating side effects. Weighing the potential benefits against the potential harms requires careful consideration of the patient's values, preferences, and overall prognosis. This delicate balance is at the heart of beneficence and non-maleficence. The physician must act as a guide, providing comprehensive information and supporting the patient's autonomy in making the best decision for themselves.

A physician's commitment to beneficence extends beyond simply prolonging life. It encompasses improving quality of life, alleviating suffering, and promoting overall well-being. This holistic approach requires a nuanced understanding of the patient's individual circumstances and priorities. For instance, for a patient with advanced cancer, the focus might shift from aggressive curative treatments to comfort care and pain management, prioritizing quality over quantity of life. This shift in priorities necessitates open communication and shared decision-making, ensuring the patient's wishes are respected and their dignity maintained. A successful outcome in such a scenario wouldn't necessarily be the patient's survival, but rather their comfort and peace of mind.

Non-maleficence, the commitment to "do no harm," is equally crucial. Medical interventions, even those intended to benefit the patient, carry inherent risks. It's the physician's responsibility to thoroughly assess these risks, balancing the potential benefits against the potential harms. This involves a detailed understanding of the procedure or treatment, including possible complications, side effects, and alternative options. Furthermore, non-maleficence extends beyond physical harm to encompass psychological and emotional well-being. A doctor's insensitive comments or a lack of empathy can inflict significant harm, undermining the patient's trust and hindering their recovery. This is particularly important to bear in mind when dealing with sensitive matters such as terminal illnesses or genetic testing results.

The principles of beneficence and non-maleficence aren't always mutually exclusive; they often intertwine in intricate ways, creating ethical dilemmas. Imagine a scenario involving a patient who refuses a life-saving blood transfusion due to religious beliefs. Respecting the patient's autonomy (as discussed in the preceding chapter) is paramount, yet the physician's commitment to beneficence compels them to advocate for the best medical outcome. This conflict highlights the need for careful consideration, open dialogue, and a thorough understanding of the patient's beliefs and values, emphasizing the collaborative nature of the doctor-patient relationship. Finding a compromise that honors both autonomy and beneficence, without causing harm, is a key goal in such situations. It also requires familiarity with relevant legal and ethical guidelines.

Applying these principles in practice frequently necessitates navigating gray areas where clear-cut answers are unavailable. The best course of action often depends on the specific context, taking into account various factors, such as the patient's age, health status, and personal beliefs. For example, aggressive treatment may be appropriate for a young patient with a high chance of recovery, but may be deemed overly burdensome for an elderly patient with a limited life expectancy. The physician's role is to guide the patient through this complex decision-making process, providing unbiased information, exploring all options, and helping them arrive at a choice aligned with their values and best interests, considering their overall well-being, not just prolonging life artificially. Open communication is instrumental to this process.

Ultimately, balancing beneficence and non-maleficence requires careful reflection, sound judgment, and a deep commitment to patient well-being. It's not merely about adhering to a set of rules but about applying ethical principles with sensitivity, empathy, and respect for the patient's autonomy. The challenges are considerable, yet the rewards – building trusting relationships, providing compassionate care, and achieving positive health outcomes – are immeasurable. The physician's responsibility extends beyond medical expertise; it embraces moral responsibility. This chapter has outlined the foundations. Consistent application, careful reflection, and continual ethical awareness are the hallmarks of true professional competence. The next chapter addresses the complex issue of justice in healthcare, further exploring the ethical framework underpinning responsible medical practice.

1.3 Justice in Healthcare

Fairness in healthcare isn't just a lofty ideal; it's a fundamental right. It demands that everyone, regardless of background or circumstance, has equal access to quality medical care. This means dismantling systemic barriers that prevent equitable distribution, ensuring healthcare isn't a privilege but a fundamental human right. We must actively fight against disparities arising from socioeconomic status, race, ethnicity, gender, sexual orientation, and geographic location. Access to healthcare is paramount, and its unequal distribution fuels a deep ethical chasm, a breach we must actively address.

The concept of justice in healthcare encompasses more than just physical access to services; it also necessitates affordability and appropriate quality of care. A system that provides expensive, inaccessible treatment to the wealthy while leaving the vulnerable behind is inherently unjust. Equitable access must therefore include affordable options, reducing financial barriers that deter crucial care. This necessitates a multi-faceted approach, including government policies, insurance reforms, and charitable initiatives to supplement or overhaul existing systems.

Consider the disparities in preventative care. Wealthier individuals often enjoy proactive health screenings and wellness programs, while those in lower socioeconomic groups frequently lack access to these essential services. This proactive approach significantly impacts long-term health outcomes, and neglecting this disparity leads to increased health complications and escalating healthcare costs. Therefore, addressing this disparity requires policies that encourage preventative care and make it readily available regardless of socioeconomic standing.

Beyond physical and financial accessibility, justice in healthcare must guarantee culturally competent care. Health professionals should provide respectful and sensitive treatment that acknowledges and addresses the cultural background and beliefs of patients. Ignoring this crucial aspect leads to poor healthcare outcomes, strained doctor-patient relationships and contributes to distrust in the healthcare system. Diversity in the healthcare workforce is key to bridging this gap and improving the quality of care for diverse populations. Training programs must emphasize cultural sensitivity to equip healthcare providers with the necessary skills to provide culturally appropriate care, improving overall care quality and inclusivity.

Furthermore, the distribution of resources within the healthcare system itself should be just. Allocation of funds, personnel, and advanced technology must prioritize areas of greatest need, not regions of affluence. We must strive for a healthcare system that actively works to address health disparities, instead of exacerbating them through uneven allocation of resources. This may involve strategic redistribution of funding, initiatives to improve healthcare infrastructure in underserved areas and the recruitment and retention of healthcare professionals in those locations.

The pursuit of justice in healthcare is a continuous process demanding ongoing commitment and vigilance. It requires a collaborative effort from healthcare professionals, policymakers, researchers, and community advocates. We must work towards ensuring fair access to high-quality healthcare for all, fostering an equitable and just healthcare system that upholds the dignity and well-being of every individual. This means critically examining current policies and practices, advocating for change and committing to ongoing improvement of the system to serve all its constituents equally. The struggle for justice in healthcare is, ultimately, a fight for human dignity and the fundamental right to health, a struggle that demands our unrelenting attention and dedicated action. The achievement of true healthcare justice will require a holistic approach, a continuous commitment to equity, and a societal shift toward prioritizing the well-being of all.

2 Chapter 2: Informed Consent

Obtaining informed consent is more than a simple signature on a form; it's the cornerstone of a trusting patient-physician relationship. Legally, it requires a competent patient, a clear explanation of the procedure, including its benefits, risks, and alternatives, and a voluntary agreement to proceed. This ensures the patient's autonomy and protects both the patient and the physician. Failure to obtain proper informed consent can lead to legal repercussions, ranging from malpractice lawsuits to disciplinary action by licensing boards. Therefore, meticulous attention to detail is crucial.

The process demands more than simply reciting a checklist. Effective communication is paramount. Employing clear, concise language, avoiding medical jargon, and tailoring explanations to the patient's understanding is crucial. Visual aids, such as diagrams or brochures, can enhance comprehension. Repeating key information and encouraging questions can further ensure understanding, allowing the patient to actively participate in the decision-making process. Remember, a truly informed decision rests on a foundation of mutual understanding.

However, the practical application presents various challenges. Patients facing complex medical issues may struggle to process the information adequately. Language barriers can further complicate the situation. Cognitive impairment, whether due to age, dementia, or other conditions, may render a patient unable to provide informed consent. In such scenarios, navigating ethical considerations requires careful attention and might necessitate seeking consent from a surrogate decision-maker, often a close family member or legal guardian. This requires sensitivity and rigorous documentation.

Dealing with patients with limited health literacy presents a significant hurdle. The complexity of medical information can be overwhelming for individuals lacking the necessary understanding of medical terminology and concepts. Therefore, adapting your communication style and employing simple, direct language become even more critical. Utilizing plain language resources, breaking down complex information into smaller, manageable chunks, and ensuring the patient understands the information before moving forward, are all vital steps. Providing written materials in an easy-to-understand format can also significantly enhance comprehension.

Situations involving minors pose unique challenges. The legal framework regarding consent for minors differs based on age and the nature of the procedure. In many cases, parental or guardian consent is required. However, the principle of assent, whereby a minor expresses their agreement to treatment, is also essential, ensuring that the minor's wishes are considered, when developmentally appropriate. This delicate balance requires a sensitive approach, ensuring the rights and perspectives of both the child and the parent or guardian are respected. Clear communication with the minor, tailored to their understanding, is critical in ensuring their cooperation and reducing fear or anxiety.

For patients who lack decision-making capacity, the process takes an even more nuanced turn. Determining incapacity requires a thorough clinical evaluation, often involving multiple professionals to assess the patient's ability to understand the information, appreciate the consequences of their decision, and weigh the risks and benefits. This evaluation should be documented meticulously, providing evidence for the decision-making process. Identifying the appropriate surrogate decision-maker, adhering to the established legal processes, and ensuring the decision aligns with the patient's best interests are paramount considerations. This requires careful consideration of ethical principles, legal standards, and cultural nuances, necessitating a multidisciplinary approach.

Beyond legal and practical challenges, the ethical dimensions of informed consent are equally significant. The physician's role extends beyond simply providing information; it involves fostering open communication and a collaborative relationship with the patient. This entails active listening, patience, and responding empathetically to the patient's concerns and questions. Building rapport and trust are essential prerequisites for securing truly informed consent. Remember that the goal is not simply to obtain consent, but to empower the patient to make an autonomous and informed decision about their own healthcare. This requires a respectful dialogue and a commitment to transparency. Effective communication underpins not only legally valid consent but also a therapeutic alliance built on trust and mutual respect, creating an environment conducive to optimal patient care.

2.1 Legal Aspects

Legal complexities significantly impact the practice of obtaining informed consent. Understanding these intricacies is paramount for physicians to avoid potential legal repercussions and maintain ethical medical practice. Negligence in obtaining proper consent can lead to malpractice lawsuits, underscoring the importance of meticulous attention to detail and thorough documentation. This extends beyond simply having a patient sign a form; it demands a comprehensive understanding of the patient's capacity for decision-making and their ability to grasp the information presented.

The legal definition of informed consent typically includes three key components: capacity, information, and voluntariness. Capacity refers to the patient's ability to understand the nature and consequences of their medical decisions. This is not solely about intelligence; factors such as age, mental illness, or the effects of medication can significantly impact a patient's capacity. Determining capacity requires careful assessment and, in certain cases, may necessitate consultation with other healthcare professionals or legal counsel. The information component encompasses providing the patient with a clear and understandable explanation of the proposed treatment, including its potential benefits, risks, and alternatives. This explanation must be tailored to the patient's level of understanding, avoiding jargon and complex medical terminology. Voluntariness ensures the patient's decision is made freely, without coercion or undue influence from family members, healthcare providers, or other external pressures. This aspect can be especially challenging when dealing with vulnerable populations or situations involving significant family dynamics.

State laws governing informed consent vary, creating a patchwork of regulations across the country. Physicians must be familiar with the specific legal requirements in their state of practice. These laws may outline specific elements that must be included in the informed consent process, such as the risks of refusing treatment, or the potential benefits of alternative treatment options. Further complicating the matter are the potential variations in court interpretations of these laws, highlighting the need for continuous professional development and staying abreast of any relevant legal updates. Failure to comply with these state-specific laws can lead to serious legal ramifications, which can range from license suspension to substantial financial penalties and even imprisonment, depending on the severity of the breach and the jurisdiction.

Documentation plays a critical role in defending against potential legal challenges. Meticulous record-keeping of the informed consent process, including the details of the conversation, the patient's questions and concerns, and any evidence demonstrating the patient's understanding, is essential. Thorough and accurate documentation serves as irrefutable evidence that the process was conducted appropriately, mitigating the risk of future legal disputes. Simply obtaining a signature on a consent form without adequate documentation of the preceding discussion does not provide sufficient legal protection. Indeed, incomplete or poorly written documentation often proves detrimental in cases involving a dispute about informed consent, and this can undermine even the most ethically sound approach to medical care.

Beyond the legal requirements, ethical considerations are inextricably interwoven with the informed consent process. While legal compliance is a minimum standard, ethical practice necessitates a commitment to fostering a true partnership with patients, actively involving them in their care decisions. Building trust and open communication is essential to ensuring that patients feel empowered to make choices that align with their values and beliefs. This process necessitates a deep understanding of the patient's personal circumstances, their health literacy, and their capacity to understand complex medical information, thereby facilitating an informed and collaborative approach. The ultimate goal is not simply legal compliance, but ethically sound and patient-centered care.

2.2 Practical Application

Obtaining truly informed consent isn't merely a matter of ticking boxes on a form. It's a dynamic process, a conversation, a careful weaving together of medical information and the patient's understanding. Consider Mrs. Rodriguez, a 72-year-old woman with limited English proficiency, facing a complex surgical procedure. Simply presenting her with a consent form in English fails to honor the principle of autonomy; she cannot truly consent without understanding the risks and benefits. Effective communication demands patience, perhaps an interpreter, and a willingness to explain the procedure in simple terms, using visual aids if necessary. Remember, genuine consent requires comprehension, not just a signature. The goal is not just legal compliance, but ethical practice. Failing to provide information in a way the patient understands undermines the very foundation of informed consent. The nuances extend beyond language. Cognitive impairment, whether due to dementia or other neurological conditions, significantly complicates the process. Imagine Mr. Jones, suffering from Alzheimer's disease, requiring a relatively minor but still invasive procedure. His capacity for decision-making may be compromised. Obtaining consent in such cases necessitates engaging family members or legal guardians, always prioritizing the patient's best interests, while acknowledging the limitations of their current cognitive abilities. Careful documentation of this process, including discussions with family members and any observations of the patient's level of understanding, is crucial in preventing future legal issues and ensuring that you've fulfilled your ethical responsibilities. Thorough record-keeping is paramount.

Beyond cognitive issues, emotional distress or coercion can also impede informed consent. A patient facing a life-threatening diagnosis might feel pressured to agree to treatment without fully understanding the implications, even if they harbor reservations. The physician's role then shifts to providing emotional support while ensuring the patient remains fully informed. Creating a safe space for questions, anxieties, and even hesitations is vital. Active listening, demonstrating empathy, and ensuring the patient feels empowered to make their own decisions are as important as the clinical information itself. Remember, the patient's emotional state can profoundly impact their ability to give truly informed consent. Patience is key.

Situations requiring urgent intervention add another layer of complexity. Imagine a trauma patient unconscious after a serious car accident. In such scenarios, the principles of beneficence and non-maleficence take precedence. While ideally, informed consent would be obtained from the patient or a designated proxy, immediate life-saving measures might be necessary before consent is possible. The ethical justification rests on the presumption that a rational person would consent to life-saving treatment in such circumstances. However, thorough documentation of the situation, the interventions taken, and subsequent efforts to contact family members or legal guardians is absolutely imperative. Transparency and open communication with the family once the patient stabilizes are vital for maintaining trust and avoiding legal repercussions. Thorough and detailed documentation safeguards against future misunderstandings.

Navigating these scenarios requires a delicate balance between legal compliance and ethical responsibility. Understanding the legal requirements is foundational; however, mere legal compliance is insufficient. The true essence of informed consent lies in fostering a collaborative relationship, empowering patients to participate actively in their healthcare decisions. Remember the human element. Treat each patient as an individual, considering their unique circumstances and capacities. Your responsibility extends beyond merely obtaining a signature; it encompasses facilitating a genuine understanding and a truly autonomous choice. The patient's voice, however faint or uncertain, needs to be heard and respected. The process should never be rushed. Effective communication is the cornerstone. These aren't just legal requirements; these are ethical imperatives.

3 Chapter 3: End-of-Life Care

Advanced directives, such as living wills and durable power of attorney for healthcare, are crucial tools for ensuring patient autonomy at the end of life. These documents allow individuals to express their wishes regarding medical treatment, should they become incapacitated and unable to make decisions for themselves. Careful consideration of these documents, involving open discussion with family and legal counsel, is paramount in respecting a patient's pre-determined choices. Ignoring or circumventing these directives can lead to significant legal and ethical complications, undermining the very principles of patient autonomy we strive to uphold. Properly executed, these directives provide clarity and guidance for healthcare providers, alleviating the burden of making life-altering decisions under immense pressure and emotional distress, enabling the focus to shift to providing optimal comfort and support to the patient.

Palliative care offers a compassionate approach to managing the symptoms of serious illnesses, focusing on improving quality of life for both the patient and their families. Unlike curative treatments, palliative care aims to relieve pain, reduce suffering, and provide emotional and spiritual support. This holistic approach encompasses physical, psychological, social, and spiritual well-being. Effective palliative care requires a multidisciplinary team, involving physicians, nurses, social workers, chaplains, and other specialists, working collaboratively to address the patient's unique needs and preferences. Moreover, it recognizes the importance of respecting patient autonomy, ensuring that treatment aligns with their values and wishes, even at the end of life. Early integration of palliative care into the treatment plan can dramatically improve the patient's comfort and experience, offering a dignified and peaceful passage.

The decision to withdraw or withhold life-sustaining treatment is often emotionally challenging but can be ethically justified when the treatment is deemed futile or excessively burdensome. Futility, in this context, refers to a situation where the treatment offers no reasonable chance of benefitting the patient, while excessive burdensomeness considers the extent of suffering the treatment causes, both physically and psychologically. These decisions necessitate careful consideration of the patient's wishes, expressed through advanced directives or family discussions, always balancing beneficence and non-maleficence. Open and honest communication with the patient and their family is crucial, ensuring mutual understanding and shared decision-making. This process should also consider the patient's overall quality of life, not just their length of life. Transparency in the decision-making process helps to alleviate anguish, promote trust, and maintain ethical integrity.

Physician-assisted suicide (PAS) and euthanasia remain highly contentious issues, eliciting intense debate among medical professionals, ethicists, and the public. PAS involves a physician providing a patient with the means to end their life, while euthanasia involves the physician directly administering a lethal substance. Both actions raise significant ethical and legal concerns, particularly regarding the potential for coercion, the slippery slope argument, and the physician's role as a healer versus an agent of death. Legal frameworks surrounding PAS and euthanasia vary considerably across jurisdictions, reflecting diverse societal values and beliefs. Regardless of legal status, physicians should engage in thorough and thoughtful reflection before considering participation in these practices, always prioritizing patient autonomy and avoiding actions that could violate their conscience or professional ethics. Furthermore, rigorous safeguards and strict regulations are crucial to minimize the risks of abuse and ensure responsible practice.

The intricacies of end-of-life care demand sensitivity, careful consideration, and a deep understanding of the ethical principles governing medical practice. It necessitates a holistic approach which balances the patient's autonomy with the physician's responsibility. Thorough knowledge of applicable laws and regulations is vital for responsible and ethical practice. Furthermore, continuous education and open dialogue among healthcare professionals are essential to navigating the complexities of these decisions and ensuring that patient care remains compassionate and respectful, even as life draws to a close. Open communication with patients and their families, ensuring clear understanding of available options, treatment implications, and the potential benefits and burdens of each, remains central. The goal, in every instance, is to alleviate suffering, promote dignity, and honor the patient's wishes, safeguarding their autonomy and ensuring a peaceful transition.

3.1 Advanced Directives

Advanced directives empower individuals to make decisions regarding their future medical care, ensuring their wishes are respected even when they lack the capacity to communicate them. These legal documents provide a crucial safeguard for patient autonomy, particularly during times of incapacitation, illness, or end-of-life situations. Understanding their significance and proper execution is essential for both healthcare professionals and the individuals they serve.

A living will, for example, allows individuals to specify the medical treatments they want or don't want to receive under specific circumstances, often focusing on life-sustaining treatments. This foresight prevents unwanted interventions and ensures a dignified end-of-life experience, aligning with the principles of beneficence and patient self-determination. Careful consideration of specific scenarios and the inclusion of detailed instructions are vital for its effectiveness. Vague statements can lead to ambiguity and potentially unwanted medical procedures.

Durable powers of attorney for healthcare delegate the authority to make medical decisions to a trusted individual, acting as the patient's surrogate decision-maker. This designated agent, often a family member or close friend, should be someone familiar with the patient's values and preferences, capable of understanding complex medical information and making decisions consistent with the patient's wishes. Choosing wisely and clearly outlining the agent's authority in the document itself is paramount. Without clear and concise instructions, the agent may face significant challenges in navigating difficult medical choices, potentially leading to conflict and distress for both the agent and family.

The execution of these documents must adhere to strict legal requirements, varying by jurisdiction. These legal requirements often include witnessing and notarization to ensure the validity and enforceability of the document. A poorly executed document may be challenged, leaving the patient's wishes vulnerable. Consulting with legal professionals familiar with healthcare law is strongly recommended to guarantee the legal soundness of the advanced directives.

Furthermore, open communication between patients, their families, and healthcare providers is vital. Discussions about end-of-life wishes and preferences are not easy, yet these conversations form the foundation of meaningful advanced directives. These conversations allow for a shared understanding of the patient's goals and values, reducing potential conflicts and promoting a more peaceful transition at life's end. Open and honest discussions can be emotionally challenging, but they are undeniably crucial for effective and ethically sound end-of-life care.

Regular review and updating of advanced directives are crucial, as life circumstances and medical advancements change. What a patient deems acceptable treatment today might change tomorrow; regularly reviewing and updating these directives ensures that they remain relevant and aligned with the individual's evolving preferences and beliefs. Failure to do so could lead to unintended consequences, potentially jeopardizing the patient's autonomy and best interests. Regular updates should be a collaborative process, involving discussions among family, the appointed agent, and possibly other trusted advisors.

Finally, understanding the limitations of advanced directives is essential. While these legal instruments are powerful tools, they cannot address every potential scenario. Some situations may require careful interpretation and thoughtful deliberation from healthcare providers, especially if the language within the advanced directives is unclear or ambiguous. Open communication and a collaborative approach among medical teams, surrogate decision-makers, and families remain pivotal to addressing such complexities while upholding the principles of patient autonomy and providing ethically sound care. These documents are tools to guide decision-making, not absolute directives.

3.2 Palliative Care

Palliative care is not about giving up; it's about embracing a different approach to treatment, one that prioritizes quality of life over aggressive interventions when a cure is no longer a realistic goal. It focuses on relieving suffering and improving the patient's overall well-being, addressing physical, emotional, and spiritual needs. This holistic perspective is crucial, acknowledging the individual's experience goes far beyond the purely medical.

The core principles of palliative care involve pain and symptom management. Effective pain control isn't just about administering medication; it's about understanding the patient's experience, their pain tolerance, and any potential side effects of the treatment. This requires a nuanced approach, regularly assessing the patient's response and adjusting the plan accordingly. Open communication with the patient and their family is vital during this process, allowing for a collaborative care plan that respects individual preferences and values.

Beyond physical comfort, palliative care addresses the emotional and psychological distress often associated with serious illness. Many patients face feelings of anxiety, depression, fear, and grief. A compassionate and supportive environment, possibly including counseling or support groups, can significantly impact their emotional well-being. The presence of family and friends offers invaluable comfort during this challenging time, and caregivers should be guided on how to provide that support effectively, minimizing the emotional burden on themselves while maximizing their contribution to the patient's well-being.

Spiritual needs also play a significant role. For many, their faith or spiritual beliefs provide strength and solace. Respecting these beliefs and integrating them into the care plan, if appropriate and desired by the patient, is crucial. This might involve connecting them with spiritual advisors or simply creating a space for reflection and prayer. It's about acknowledging the patient's complete being and allowing them to experience comfort in their own ways.

Furthermore, palliative care isn't solely for the dying patient; it can be offered concurrently with curative treatments. For instance, a cancer patient undergoing chemotherapy might also receive palliative care to manage their pain, nausea, and fatigue. This combined approach maximizes the patient's overall quality of life throughout their journey. It demonstrates the crucial role of palliative care as a complementary approach, extending its benefit to a much wider spectrum of patients than often presumed.

Effective palliative care requires a multidisciplinary team approach. Physicians, nurses, social workers, chaplains, and other specialists work together to provide comprehensive care. This collaborative effort ensures all aspects of the patient's needs are addressed. Clear communication and coordination among team members are essential, especially concerning end-of-life decision-making, ensuring clarity and coherence in actions taken.

Finally, the ethical considerations within palliative care are paramount. Respecting patient autonomy is fundamental, ensuring the patient's wishes, preferences, and values are central to the care plan. This includes respecting their right to refuse treatment, even if it might lead to a shorter lifespan. It's about empowering the patient to make informed choices about their own care journey, making their final moments meaningful and in alignment with their own values. Balancing beneficence (acting in the patient's best interest) and respecting autonomy often requires careful judgment and sensitive conversations.

3.3 Withdrawing Treatment

Withdrawing life-sustaining treatment is a profoundly complex decision, fraught with ethical and emotional weight. It's a process that requires careful consideration of the patient's wishes, their medical prognosis, and the potential consequences of both continuing and discontinuing treatment. We've already covered informed consent; now, we must focus on its practical application in this incredibly sensitive area. This isn't simply about turning off a machine; it's about navigating a labyrinth of legal, ethical, and human considerations to ensure the patient's dignity and autonomy are respected.

The legal landscape surrounding withdrawing treatment is complex and varies significantly depending on jurisdiction. In many places, competent adults have the right to refuse any medical treatment, even if that refusal leads to their death. This right is firmly rooted in the principle of autonomy—the patient's right to self-determination regarding their own body and medical care. However, this right isn't absolute. It becomes particularly challenging when the patient lacks the capacity to make decisions for themselves, either due to cognitive impairment or a lack of consciousness. In such cases, surrogate decision-makers, typically family members, step in to act in the patient's best interests, relying on previously expressed wishes, if any, or making judgments based on what they believe the patient would have wanted. This process can be emotionally wrenching for everyone involved.

Navigating these legal complexities often requires close collaboration between medical professionals, the patient (or their surrogate), and potentially legal counsel. Clear and open communication is paramount. Doctors need to explain the patient's condition, the available treatment options, and the potential consequences of each, including the likely outcome of withdrawing treatment. They must also ensure that the patient—or their designated surrogate—fully understands the information and has the opportunity to ask questions and express concerns. This is not a moment for rushed decisions; careful deliberation is crucial for the doctor's and patient's conscience alike.

The ethical dimensions of withdrawing treatment are equally multifaceted. The principle of beneficence, acting in the patient's best interest, often comes into conflict with the principle of non-maleficence, avoiding harm. Continuing futile treatment, for example, might prolong suffering without offering any real benefit, thereby constituting harm. In these situations, carefully weighing the potential benefits and harms is essential. Furthermore, maintaining the patient's dignity throughout the process is paramount. This includes providing comfort, pain relief, and emotional support, whether treatment is continued or withdrawn. Ultimately, the goal is to ensure the patient's death, if it occurs, is as peaceful and respectful as possible.

Ethical considerations also extend to the healthcare team. Physicians and nurses involved in the decision-making process may struggle with emotional distress. The potential for moral conflict is significant, especially when there are disagreements about the best course of action. Providing access to support services for the healthcare team, including emotional support and ethical consultation, is therefore crucial. It is vital to recognize the psychological toll on those who must navigate these immensely difficult situations. Open and honest conversations within the healthcare team, as well as external consultations, can help alleviate potential emotional burden and ensure the process adheres to the highest ethical standards. The professional support systems available to doctors need to acknowledge the emotional weight of this decision-making.

The practical implications of withdrawing treatment often involve the careful titration of medications, the removal of life-sustaining equipment, or both. These actions must be carried out with the utmost care and sensitivity, ensuring the patient's comfort and dignity are preserved. Pain management and symptom control should be a priority to minimize suffering. Furthermore, close monitoring of the patient's condition is necessary after treatment is withdrawn to ensure a peaceful transition, providing both family and medical team with a sense of control and security. Palliative care, as discussed in a prior chapter, will play a crucial role in this final phase.

In conclusion, withdrawing treatment is a serious decision with profound ethical, legal, and practical implications. It demands a careful consideration of the patient's autonomy, best interests, and the potential harms of both continuing and withdrawing treatment. Open communication, collaborative decision-making, and compassion are essential throughout the process. The ultimate aim is to navigate this difficult situation with sensitivity, respect, and a commitment to upholding both patient autonomy and the highest standards of medical ethics. The emotional well-being of both the patient and the medical team should be paramount, guiding every step of this delicate procedure. Every individual involved deserves to receive unwavering support through this complex period.

3.4 Physician-Assisted Suicide

Physician-assisted suicide (PAS) occupies a uniquely fraught space within end-of-life care. Its very existence sparks intense debate, pitting deeply held beliefs about the sanctity of life against the equally compelling principle of patient autonomy. The central question, consistently debated and redefined, remains: when, if ever, does a physician's responsibility extend to actively assisting a patient's death? This is not a simple question, and ethical considerations are paramount. The nuances require careful consideration of the patient's suffering, the availability of palliative care, and the potential for coercion or abuse.

The legal landscape surrounding PAS is far from uniform. Some jurisdictions have legalized it under tightly regulated conditions, mandating rigorous evaluations of the patient's mental capacity, prognosis, and the absence of any treatable underlying conditions that could improve their quality of life. These laws often include safeguards like multiple physician consultations and waiting periods, designed to minimize the risk of hasty or ill-considered decisions. Such regulations, however, remain controversial, with some arguing that they fail to adequately protect vulnerable individuals. In many places, PAS remains entirely illegal, prompting discussions of access to end-of-life care for patients in situations of unbearable suffering. Many physicians find themselves deeply conflicted by the prospect of participating in PAS. While embracing patient autonomy, their inherent commitment to preserving life can create a powerful internal struggle. This is compounded by the professional risk, and ethical implications involved, creating a need for robust support systems for those grappling with these decisions. The decision to participate, or not, is deeply personal and should be made conscientiously, with careful consideration of one's own ethical framework and the specific context of each case. For physicians, the emotional toll can be substantial, potentially requiring access to specialized counseling or support groups to ensure their wellbeing.

Conversely, for patients facing terminal illness and intractable suffering, the choice of PAS can offer a sense of agency and control over their final moments. The ability to make this decision, within a framework of informed consent and appropriate safeguards, is vital for respecting their autonomy. The experience of prolonged, unbearable suffering can have a profound impact on an individual's dignity and sense of self, and the opportunity to choose a peaceful, controlled exit can be seen as a crucial aspect of end-of-life care. The challenge lies in ensuring that this choice is genuinely free from coercion, reflecting the patient's true wishes and understanding of the available alternatives.

Furthermore, the discussion around PAS invariably touches upon the issue of access to palliative care. Adequate pain management and symptom control can dramatically improve the quality of life for those in the final stages of life, potentially diminishing the desire for PAS. Investing in robust palliative care programs, accessible to all, is essential for offering a comprehensive alternative to PAS. By providing comprehensive comfort and support, palliative care aims to alleviate physical and emotional suffering, allowing patients to focus on their relationships and spiritual well-being. It's the ethical duty of the medical profession to assure the availability of these vital services, thereby lessening the need for PAS as a response to unbearable suffering.

Finally, the ongoing debate surrounding PAS highlights the inherent complexity of ethical decision-making in healthcare. The need to balance patient autonomy with the physician's responsibility to preserve life necessitates a nuanced and compassionate approach. Ongoing dialogue among healthcare professionals, ethicists, policymakers, and the public is crucial to clarifying the parameters of PAS, safeguarding against potential abuses, and ensuring that those facing life-limiting illnesses are treated with dignity and respect. This includes examining access to care, the training of healthcare providers, and the establishment of clear guidelines that balance patient rights with ethical considerations of medical practice. The continued exploration of these aspects will shape the future of end-of-life care.

3.5 Euthanasia

Euthanasia is a deeply complex issue, stirring intense emotions and philosophical debate. It's a topic that necessitates careful consideration of patient autonomy, the physician's role, and the broader societal implications. While previous chapters have explored patient autonomy and the ethical framework guiding medical practice, euthanasia demands a specific focus, acknowledging the unique circumstances and profound moral weight involved. We must approach this with sensitivity and a deep understanding of the multifaceted ethical challenges.

The central ethical dilemma revolves around the patient's right to self-determination versus the physician's obligation to preserve life. Advocates for euthanasia emphasize the importance of respecting a terminally ill patient's wish to end their suffering, arguing that denying this choice infringes upon their autonomy and dignity. This argument is particularly poignant when considering unbearable pain and a severely diminished quality of life. The concept of bodily autonomy, firmly established in other medical contexts, is directly relevant here. However, this is where it gets nuanced and complex.

Conversely, opponents often cite the sanctity of life, arguing that intentionally ending a life, even at the patient's request, is morally wrong. Religious and philosophical beliefs frequently underpin this perspective. Furthermore, concerns exist regarding the potential for coercion or abuse, particularly for vulnerable patients who might feel pressured to choose euthanasia even if they don't truly desire it.

The slippery slope argument, warning of potential unintended consequences and expansion of the practice beyond its intended limits, is often raised.

The legal landscape surrounding euthanasia varies dramatically across jurisdictions globally. In some places, it's explicitly permitted under strict guidelines, often requiring multiple evaluations and a clear demonstration of the patient's informed consent, along with their irremediable suffering. In other regions, euthanasia remains illegal, despite the existence of related practices such as physician-assisted suicide, which is a slightly different, yet equally intricate topic. A thorough comprehension of the legal framework in one's specific location is indispensable for navigating this ethically fraught terrain.

Consider the case of a patient suffering from a debilitating, incurable illness, experiencing constant and unbearable pain. Their quality of life is drastically diminished. They've expressed a clear, persistent wish to end their suffering, demonstrating full comprehension of the implications. Their family supports this decision, recognizing the depth of their pain and their desire for peace. However, the physician has personal or religious objections to euthanasia. This presents a considerable conflict – the physician's personal beliefs versus the patient's autonomous choice.

The role of palliative care becomes critically important in these scenarios. While not a direct solution to the euthanasia debate, high-quality palliative care aims to alleviate suffering, enhance quality of life, and provide emotional support. A holistic approach, considering physical, psychological, and spiritual needs, can greatly reduce the desire for euthanasia. Indeed, many patients, once provided with comprehensive palliative care, may find that their suffering is manageable and their desire for euthanasia diminished or disappears entirely. This is a very crucial element to consider.

Ultimately, the decision regarding euthanasia is a deeply personal one, demanding thoughtful consideration from all parties involved. While medical professionals play a vital role in providing information, support, and care, the final choice should rest with the patient. However, maintaining the highest ethical standards throughout this process is imperative. This means ensuring informed consent, excluding coercion, and providing access to appropriate resources, such as palliative care and counseling. The conversation itself must be handled with utmost care and sensitivity. It isn't merely about the technicalities of medical procedures; it involves facing profound existential questions, grappling with profound losses, and accepting the inevitability of death. Navigating these complexities requires a delicate balance between respecting patient autonomy and fulfilling the physician's ethical responsibilities. The physician's role is not to judge, but to listen, counsel, and guide, offering compassion and support to both the patient and their loved ones. The complexity of the subject matters and the legal aspects differ profoundly depending on the location, therefore, local laws and regulations must be carefully considered.

4 Chapter 4: Resource Allocation

Healthcare resources, sadly, are not infinite. This fundamental truth presents healthcare professionals with some of the most challenging ethical dilemmas imaginable. We strive for beneficence, to always act in the best interests of our patients, yet limited resources often force difficult choices, demanding prioritization and, inevitably, the rationing of care. This chapter explores the complex world of resource allocation, examining the ethical frameworks we can use to navigate these agonizing decisions.

The scarcity of resources isn't just a theoretical problem; it's a daily reality in many healthcare settings. Consider the limited number of organ transplant slots, the finite supply of expensive medications, or the overburdened capacity of intensive care units. These are not abstract concepts; these are real situations with real consequences for patients' lives. These limitations demand a robust and ethical approach to decision-making.

Several ethical frameworks can guide us in these trying circumstances. Utilitarianism, for instance, suggests that we should allocate resources in a way that maximizes overall benefit for the greatest number of people. This approach, while seemingly straightforward, can lead to incredibly difficult choices, potentially sacrificing the well-being of some individuals for the benefit of many. Weighing potential benefits against the potential harms is a constant struggle.

A contrasting approach emphasizes the principle of equity. This framework champions equal distribution of resources, regardless of individual circumstances or potential outcomes. While morally appealing, ensuring perfect equity in a world of limited resources is practically impossible, given that needs and circumstances vary so widely among patients. It's a worthy ideal, but requires careful consideration and a nuanced approach.

A third framework, often used in combination with others, emphasizes the concept of need. This prioritizes patients with the most urgent or severe medical needs, regardless of factors like cost-effectiveness or prognosis. This approach prioritizes the immediate relief of suffering, though it risks neglecting preventive care and long-term health benefits. Ultimately, decisions often demand careful evaluation of all three approaches together, leading to a balanced and comprehensive strategy.

Moreover, the allocation process itself needs to be transparent and accountable. Clear, well-defined criteria, regularly reviewed and updated based on evidence and expert opinions, are essential. This transparency builds trust with patients and the public, fostering understanding and acceptance, even when decisions are difficult. Without clear parameters and ongoing evaluation, resource allocation processes risk appearing arbitrary and unjust.

The concept of cost-effectiveness often enters the discussion. While aiming for the most cost-effective treatments is important for resource management, prioritizing cost above all other factors can lead to ethically questionable decisions. For example, denying a life-saving treatment simply because it's expensive can be deemed unethical, as healthcare is not merely a commodity; it is a fundamental human right.

However, ignoring cost entirely is also impractical. Resource allocation requires a delicate balance between ethical considerations and economic realities. A sustainable healthcare system must make the most efficient use of available resources, without compromising ethical standards. We are constantly walking a tightrope.

Beyond individual cases, ethical resource allocation requires considering broader societal impacts. Investing in preventive care, for instance, can prevent many future illnesses, reducing the overall burden on healthcare resources. Likewise, addressing social determinants of health – poverty, inequality, and lack of access to education

– can significantly improve overall health and reduce the demand for costly interventions down the line. Addressing social inequality is a major key to improving health outcomes.

Ultimately, resource allocation is not simply a matter of applying a formula or algorithm. It's a deeply human endeavor, requiring empathy, careful consideration of ethical principles, and a commitment to fairness and justice. While there are no easy answers, it's imperative for healthcare professionals to engage in open discussions, rely on transparent processes, and prioritize ethical considerations in all aspects of decision-making. Each situation necessitates a thoughtful, case-by-case evaluation, prioritizing empathy, fairness, and adherence to ethical guidelines. These are not merely abstract concepts but rather practical tools that shape the core of the healthcare system. The responsibility of appropriate resource allocation is not only a moral obligation but also a vital aspect of creating a just and equitable healthcare system.

4.1 Scarcity & Prioritization

Healthcare resources are finite. This inherent scarcity forces difficult choices, demanding a systematic approach to prioritization that balances ethical principles with practical realities. We can't provide everything to everyone, a stark truth demanding careful consideration. The ethical weight of these decisions rests heavily on healthcare professionals, requiring a nuanced understanding of the principles guiding resource allocation.

Prioritization isn't arbitrary. It involves a multifaceted assessment of patient needs, weighing the potential benefits of interventions against their costs, both financial and otherwise. This includes considering the severity of illness, the likelihood of successful treatment, and the patient's overall prognosis. It's a complex equation, lacking easy answers, and often involving difficult trade-offs. Consider a scenario where two patients require a limited supply of a life-saving medication. One patient has a higher chance of recovery, while the other's condition is more critical.

The choice becomes agonizing.

Utilitarian principles suggest maximizing overall benefit, potentially favoring the patient with the greater chance of survival and long-term health. This approach aims to achieve the greatest good for the greatest number, but it's not without its critics, leading to concerns of potential biases. Justice demands fair and equitable distribution, regardless of individual circumstances. This means avoiding discrimination based on factors like age, socioeconomic status, or race. Striking a balance between these two competing values is a key challenge in resource allocation.

Transparency is crucial. Openly discussing resource limitations and the rationale behind prioritization decisions with patients and their families fosters trust and understanding. It allows them to participate actively in decisions concerning their care, acknowledging the constraints imposed by the system. This transparency might not alleviate the pain of difficult choices but it can promote a sense of shared responsibility and mitigate resentment.

Establishing clear guidelines and protocols for resource allocation is essential. These guidelines should be developed collaboratively with input from ethicists, healthcare professionals, and the community. Their implementation must be regularly reviewed and adapted to evolving circumstances. Consistent application of these protocols not only minimizes bias but also ensures accountability and transparency in the decision-making process. This process avoids arbitrary decisions made on the spur of the moment and allows for systematic review and potential refinement over time.

The development of these guidelines is never a finished project. Healthcare needs and available resources constantly evolve, and our understanding of disease and treatment options shifts as well. Consequently, ethical frameworks for resource allocation must be regularly reviewed and revised to ensure their continued relevance and applicability. This dynamic process acknowledges the complexity of the subject and demands a constant re-evaluation of the principles and practices involved. Continuous professional development is vital for healthcare professionals in adapting to these developments and making informed decisions.

Furthermore, the societal impact of scarcity demands attention. Investing in preventative healthcare and health promotion programs can reduce the overall demand for scarce resources. Addressing underlying social determinants of health, like poverty and inequality, can also have a significant impact on reducing health disparities. These are preventative measures that mitigate the need for drastic prioritization in the long run.

Finally, remember that prioritization is not just about allocating scarce resources, it's about providing compassionate and ethical care. Every interaction with a patient should be guided by the principles of beneficence, non-maleficence, and respect for autonomy. This means recognizing the limits of medical intervention and providing holistic care that attends to the physical, emotional, and spiritual needs of the individual. It is crucial that the entire system upholds the value of every human life, regardless of access to resources. While scarcity necessitates choices, compassion should always be at the heart of medical decision making. The ethical considerations surrounding resource allocation are multifaceted and complex, requiring continuous reflection, adaptation and collaboration from both healthcare professionals and the broader community.

4.2 Ethical Dilemmas

Limited healthcare resources force difficult choices. Imagine a scenario: two patients, both critically ill, require the same scarce organ for transplant. One is a young mother with a bright future, the other an elderly patient nearing the end of life. Who receives the organ? This seemingly simple question unveils a complex web of ethical dilemmas demanding careful consideration of competing values. Prioritizing based solely on age is ethically questionable, disregarding the value of each life. A purely utilitarian approach, maximizing the number of years of life saved, would favor the younger patient, but ignores the quality of life remaining for both. The ethical framework outlined earlier offers guidance but provides no easy answers. The inherent tension between beneficence – the desire to do good – and justice –

ensuring fair distribution – becomes starkly apparent. This forces us to consider not only the immediate impact on the patients, but the long-term implications of our decisions on healthcare policy and the allocation of resources. We must constantly re-evaluate our approach, remaining mindful of the societal impact of our choices.

The principle of justice demands equitable access to healthcare, regardless of social standing, wealth, or other factors unrelated to medical need. However, the reality of limited resources forces difficult prioritization decisions. We are forced to confront the agonizing question of how to fairly distribute scarce resources, a task that is far from straightforward. A transparent and well-defined system, open to public scrutiny and regularly reviewed, is crucial. This system must allow for the consideration of both individual patient needs and the overall well-being of the community, balancing the seemingly irreconcilable. It might incorporate several factors, including prognosis, severity of illness, potential benefit from treatment, and even the patient's own expressed wishes, whenever possible. The key is to strive for a process that is both justifiable and as fair as possible within the constraints of the situation. The constant tension between individual rights and the needs of the community as a whole remains at the heart of this dilemma.

Consider the role of cost-effectiveness analysis in resource allocation. This approach objectively evaluates different treatment options based on their effectiveness and cost, guiding decisions toward the most efficient uses of scarce funds. Yet, solely focusing on cost-effectiveness might lead to ethically questionable outcomes. It could lead to the prioritization of treatments with high cost-effectiveness ratios, potentially overlooking the needs of individuals with conditions that, while less cost-effective, are nevertheless life-saving or improve quality of life significantly. A purely cost-effective approach can devalue lives considered "less valuable" from a purely economic viewpoint, creating an ethically problematic system. Striking a balance between economic efficiency and the ethical imperative to ensure equitable access remains a continuing challenge. The solution, likely, lies not in a single metric, but in a careful, thoughtful integration of factors, with constant ethical review and scrutiny.

Furthermore, considering the patient's perspective significantly influences ethical decision-making. Individual autonomy demands that patients are fully informed and involved in choices affecting their care, even in situations of limited resources. This includes giving patients the opportunity to express their preferences and values, even if these choices seem less medically efficient. Of course, respecting autonomy doesn't mean acquiescing to every wish, but it does mean actively engaging patients in the decision-making process. This process requires empathy, clear communication, and a genuine effort to understand the patient's unique perspective and concerns. It is crucial to not only focus on the medical facts, but also the patient's overall wellbeing, their anxieties, and their life goals and values. Only in such way can the physician truly assist the patient in making the most informed choice, even within the constraints of resource limitations.

Ethical dilemmas surrounding resource allocation are not merely abstract theoretical challenges; they represent real-world situations with profound consequences for both patients and healthcare professionals. The complexities involved demand a nuanced approach that combines rigorous ethical principles, clinical expertise, and a deep respect for the inherent dignity and value of each individual life. The goal is not to eliminate these challenges, which are inherent in the human experience, but to navigate them ethically and thoughtfully, always striving to ensure the fairest and most compassionate care possible. Each situation is unique, demanding careful and individualized attention. The guiding principle should always be to act in the best interest of the patient, while maintaining a commitment to fairness and equity for all.

5 Chapter 5: Medical Error & Disclosure

Medical errors, sadly, are an unavoidable reality in healthcare. Despite the best intentions and rigorous training, mistakes happen. The crucial element isn't avoiding errors entirely – that's an unrealistic goal – but rather how we respond when they occur. Our response defines the integrity of our profession and significantly impacts the patient's healing journey. Transparency and honesty are paramount.

A culture of blame and cover-ups only exacerbates the situation, hindering learning and preventing future incidents. Openly acknowledging mistakes fosters trust and allows for a more collaborative approach to rectifying the situation and preventing similar occurrences. This collaborative approach includes involving the patient in the process, making them an active participant in their own care. Failing to acknowledge an error can lead to a severe erosion of trust, potentially damaging the physician-patient relationship beyond repair. This damage is not merely emotional but can have significant legal consequences.

The legal ramifications of undisclosed medical errors are substantial. Patients have the right to know about any medical mistake that has affected their treatment. Withholding this information can lead to malpractice lawsuits, disciplinary actions from licensing boards, and reputational damage. These consequences extend beyond the individual physician, affecting the entire healthcare system. Open communication and full disclosure, while challenging, ultimately serve to protect both the patient and the physician. Furthermore, legal precedents strongly support the ethical duty to disclose medical errors. Transparency isn't just the 'right thing to do'; it's often legally mandated. The lack of disclosure often signifies a lack of commitment to patient welfare, a disregard for ethical responsibilities, and a neglect of professional accountability.

Effective communication with the patient is at the heart of appropriate disclosure. This requires empathy, sensitivity, and a genuine commitment to providing the patient with the necessary information to understand what happened, the impact on their health, and the steps being taken to address the error and minimize further harm. The conversation should not be a sterile recitation of facts; it should be a dialogue that acknowledges the patient's emotions, validates their concerns, and provides them with realistic and transparent expectations of the course of recovery. This requires an understanding of what constitutes effective communication, considering various factors, such as the patient's emotional and cognitive state, their preferred communication style, and the cultural context of the interaction.

The process should also involve detailing the steps being taken to prevent similar errors from recurring. This demonstrates a commitment to continuous improvement within the healthcare setting, underscoring a proactive approach to risk management. Such proactive measures, including improved protocols, enhanced training, and increased oversight, are crucial not just for legal protection but also for maintaining the highest standards of patient safety. This is a vital component of maintaining public trust in the medical profession. The focus should be on learning from the mistake, improving processes and procedures to reduce the risk of future occurrences. Transparency, in this context, is not just about admitting fault; it's about demonstrating responsibility and commitment to continuous quality improvement.

Addressing errors head-on, with genuine remorse and a proactive plan for addressing the situation and preventing recurrence, is paramount for maintaining trust and fostering a healthy physician-patient relationship. The emotional toll on both the patient and the physician should be acknowledged and addressed appropriately. The patient's experience is central, and validating their emotions is key to a productive and healing interaction. This isn't simply a legal formality; it's a human interaction requiring empathy, honesty, and a commitment to healing. Effective communication requires not only clear articulation of the facts but also sensitivity to the emotional impact on the patient, their family, and the involved healthcare providers. Providing appropriate support, whether through referral to counseling services or other assistance, demonstrates a genuine concern for the well-being of those affected.

Finally, remember that the disclosure process isn't solely about the legal implications; it's fundamentally about ethical responsibility. It's about upholding the trust that underpins the doctor-patient relationship. It's about owning our actions and contributing to the improvement of the healthcare system. Mistakes will occur; how we respond to those mistakes ultimately defines our commitment to the ethical principles that guide our profession, emphasizing the ongoing pursuit of excellence in patient care and safety. This is a critical aspect of both maintaining the trust of patients and demonstrating commitment to ongoing professional improvement and responsibility. The focus must always remain on placing patient welfare and well-being above all else. The commitment to ethical conduct, even amidst unforeseen challenges, remains the cornerstone of a strong and credible medical profession.

5.1 Transparency & Trust

Open communication is paramount. Transparency, in the context of medical errors, isn't simply about admitting fault; it's about rebuilding trust, a cornerstone of the doctor-patient relationship, often fractured by unforeseen complications. This isn't about blame; it's about shared understanding and a collaborative path forward, focusing on the patient's recovery and well-being. A frank discussion, even when difficult, fosters healing and prevents future misunderstandings, fostering a stronger, more resilient bond.

Immediate and honest disclosure is crucial. Delaying the conversation breeds mistrust and suspicion, allowing speculation to fester. Prompt communication, however painful, demonstrates respect for the patient's autonomy and their right to know. It's also legally prudent, mitigating potential lawsuits and ensuring compliance with medical standards. Think about the relief you'd feel knowing the truth, rather than being left in the dark to grapple with uncertainty.

A sincere apology, while acknowledging the mistake, needs to be carefully worded. Avoid language that might be interpreted as evasive or dismissive. Phrases like "I'm so sorry this happened" are generally better than more impersonal statements. The focus should remain on the patient's experience and their concerns, rather than on assigning blame or making excuses. Remember, empathy and genuine remorse are more effective than technical explanations.

Detailed explanation of the error is essential, but remember your audience. Use clear and concise language, avoiding medical jargon that might be confusing or alienating. Focus on what occurred, the potential consequences, and the steps you've taken to prevent similar incidents. Visual aids, if appropriate, can enhance understanding and facilitate open dialogue, creating a safe space for your patients to feel they are heard.

A collaborative plan for recovery is fundamental. This goes beyond immediate treatment. It includes discussing long-term effects, rehabilitation options, and ongoing monitoring. Involve the patient in this process, allowing them to make informed decisions about their care, demonstrating respect for their self-determination. This partnership, built on trust, is more likely to lead to a successful outcome.

Active listening is pivotal. Patients need to feel heard, not just listened to. Pay close attention to their emotional state, addressing concerns and fears openly and compassionately. Allow them to express their emotions without interruption, even if they're angry or upset. This demonstration of emotional intelligence strengthens the therapeutic alliance and promotes healing.

Documentation is vital. Maintain a comprehensive record of the error, the disclosure conversation, and the subsequent steps taken. This detailed documentation will help ensure accountability and assist in identifying areas for improvement within the healthcare system. It also serves as a legal safeguard, providing evidence of your transparency and commitment to patient well-being. This is not just about protection; it's about continuous learning and improvement.

Learning from mistakes is essential. Errors are inevitable in medicine, but a commitment to learning from them is crucial. Analyze what went wrong, discuss this with colleagues, and implement changes to prevent similar incidents. This commitment to continuous improvement is a key element in fostering trust and demonstrating responsibility to the profession, and most importantly, your patients. This demonstrates a proactive approach, valuing patient safety above all else.

Building trust takes time. Even after full disclosure and remediation, rebuilding trust requires ongoing effort. Maintain open communication, promptly address any concerns, and be consistently responsive to your patients' needs. Regular follow-up appointments, empathetic listening, and a sincere commitment to their well-being are all essential components of restoring and maintaining trust.

The healing process transcends the immediate medical issue. It involves restoring the patient's faith in the healthcare system and in their physician. Remember, your role isn't solely limited to the physical; the emotional and psychological aspects of care are paramount. Prioritizing empathy and understanding in every interaction strengthens the bond and fosters trust. The relationship is the cornerstone of successful healthcare. Transparency and trust are more than just concepts, they're the foundation for high-quality, ethical medical care.

5.2 Legal Ramifications

Medical errors, while regrettable, are an unavoidable reality in healthcare. Their occurrence, however, doesn't negate the physician's responsibility; rather, it necessitates a transparent and ethically sound response. Failing to acknowledge and address errors can have significant legal repercussions, potentially leading to malpractice lawsuits and damage to one's professional reputation. Open communication is paramount—not only does it foster trust with the patient, but it also demonstrates a commitment to patient well-being and professional accountability. The legal landscape surrounding medical errors is complex and varies by jurisdiction, encompassing aspects like negligence, breach of duty, and proximate cause. Understanding these legal nuances is crucial for safeguarding oneself and acting responsibly.

A crucial element in managing the legal ramifications of medical errors is comprehensive documentation. Meticulous record-keeping, including detailed descriptions of procedures, patient assessments, and any complications encountered, serves as a robust defense against potential legal challenges. Documentation should accurately reflect the care provided and any unforeseen circumstances. Moreover, diligent adherence to established medical protocols and guidelines significantly reduces the risk of errors and strengthens a legal position should disputes arise. Remember, the goal isn't to avoid accountability, but to demonstrate responsible practice and a commitment to patient safety. It is imperative to consult with legal counsel specializing in medical malpractice to stay abreast of relevant laws and best practices for managing potential litigation.

Beyond the immediate legal implications, the emotional toll on both the physician and the patient cannot be ignored. Medical errors often trigger feelings of guilt, shame, and self-doubt in the physician, impacting their mental health and professional confidence. Simultaneously, the patient and their family may experience a range of emotions, including anger, betrayal, and grief. Supporting the patient through this difficult time is crucial, and often involves addressing not just the physical aspects of the injury or illness, but also the emotional and psychological ones. Open and honest communication, even in the face of difficult news, can help build trust and prevent the escalation of resentment. Seeking support from colleagues, mentors, or professionals in mental health can aid in processing the emotional aftermath of a medical error.

The legal system offers various avenues for resolution beyond formal litigation. Mediation and arbitration, for instance, provide alternative dispute resolution methods that can be more efficient and less adversarial. These methods can help resolve conflicts, reduce financial burdens associated with litigation, and preserve professional relationships. The availability of these options varies by jurisdiction and the nature of the dispute. The decision to pursue such alternative methods often relies on the specific facts of the case, the preferences of all parties involved, and the guidance of legal counsel. The primary goal should always remain centered on patient well-being and fair resolution.

Ultimately, preventing medical errors should be the primary focus. This involves implementing robust systems for quality improvement, fostering a culture of safety within medical institutions, and prioritizing ongoing medical education and training. Continuous self-reflection and a commitment to evidence-based practice can significantly reduce the likelihood of errors. Furthermore, teamwork and open communication among healthcare professionals are paramount in identifying and mitigating potential risks. A proactive approach to risk management minimizes the likelihood of legal ramifications while simultaneously demonstrating a commitment to the highest standards of patient care. Regular review of protocols, equipment, and staffing levels, combined with consistent adherence to safety guidelines, is essential in minimizing the potential for future errors and therefore, future legal battles.

The landscape of medical malpractice claims is continuously evolving, influenced by factors such as technological advancements, changes in healthcare regulations, and shifts in public perception. Staying informed about the latest legal precedents, best practices, and emerging trends is critical for all healthcare professionals. Participation in professional organizations, ongoing continuing medical education (CME) courses, and regular consultation with legal experts specializing in medical law can help physicians navigate the complexities of the legal environment and ensure that they are practicing within acceptable legal boundaries. This proactive approach not only safeguards individual careers, but also helps to maintain the integrity and credibility of the medical profession as a whole. Remember, responsible practice is not just ethically sound; it's also legally prudent.

The emotional and psychological impact of a medical error is often overlooked. It is imperative to remember that physicians are human, and mistakes happen. It's vital to have a support system in place to help navigate the emotional fallout of such events. Seeking professional guidance from counselors or therapists specializing in physician well-being is highly advisable. This helps to process the stress, grief, or guilt experienced and to maintain a healthy perspective. Openly discussing challenges with colleagues or mentors can provide valuable support and help to prevent isolation, which can further exacerbate the emotional strain. It is equally important to approach patients and families with empathy and compassion, acknowledging the suffering caused by the error and focusing on collaborative efforts to rectify the situation and provide appropriate care.

The ethical and legal aspects of medical error disclosure are interconnected and must be carefully considered. While transparency is essential for building trust with patients and maintaining ethical integrity, the manner in which information is disclosed must be handled with great care. It's crucial to consult with legal counsel to ensure that all legal requirements are met and to develop a communication strategy that balances honesty with patient well-being. The goal is not only to disclose the error but also to offer genuine apologies, explain the steps being taken to prevent future occurrences, and to address the patient's concerns in a compassionate and constructive way. Careful consideration must be given to the potential for the disclosure to impact the patient's emotional well-being and how to best mitigate any potential adverse effects. A compassionate approach should always be coupled with legal prudence.

In conclusion, while medical errors are a potential source of significant legal ramifications, proactive risk management strategies, open communication, comprehensive documentation, and a supportive professional environment can significantly reduce the likelihood of adverse legal consequences. Remembering that responsible practice is both ethically and legally sound is paramount. Continuous learning, consistent adherence to best practices, and a willingness to accept accountability are not just markers of professionalism; they are essential for protecting oneself and maintaining the integrity of the medical profession. By actively fostering a culture of safety and transparency, and understanding the legal frameworks governing medical errors, physicians can ensure that they are not only providing the best possible patient care, but also safeguarding their own professional well-being. Prioritizing patient safety and maintaining open communication are not merely good practices—they are legal necessities.

5.3 Patient Communication

Effective communication is the cornerstone of a strong physician-patient relationship, crucial for navigating the complexities of modern healthcare. It's not merely about conveying information; it's about building trust, fostering understanding, and empowering patients to participate actively in their care. This requires more than just technical skill; it demands empathy, active listening, and a genuine commitment to patient-centered care. Ignoring these fundamental aspects can lead to misunderstandings, decreased adherence to treatment plans, and even legal repercussions.

The art of patient communication hinges on several key elements. First and foremost is active listening. This goes beyond simply hearing the patient's words; it involves paying close attention to their nonverbal cues, such as body language and tone of voice, to gain a holistic understanding of their concerns. It requires patience, a willingness to set aside preconceived notions, and a genuine desire to understand the patient's perspective, even if it differs from your own. Remember to summarize and reflect back their points to confirm understanding and encourage further discussion.

A crucial aspect of effective communication lies in tailoring your approach to the individual patient. Consider their age, cultural background, educational level, and emotional state when conveying information. Use clear, concise language, avoiding medical jargon that may confuse or intimidate them. Visual aids such as diagrams or pamphlets can be invaluable tools for enhancing comprehension, especially for complex medical conditions. Always ensure you're speaking at a pace they can understand and consistently check for comprehension. A simple "Do you understand?" can make a significant difference.

Open-ended questions are essential to encourage patients to express their thoughts and feelings freely. Avoid leading questions that may inadvertently influence their responses. Instead, promote a dialogue where patients feel comfortable expressing doubts, concerns, or even anxieties about their treatment plan. This open communication is essential for addressing potential misconceptions and building trust. Remember you're dealing with more than just the disease, you're dealing with a whole person with emotional responses to health issues.

Transparency is paramount in building trust. Patients have a right to accurate, honest information about their diagnosis, prognosis, treatment options, and potential risks and benefits. While delivering difficult news can be challenging, it's imperative to do so with compassion, empathy, and sensitivity. Allow space for questions, answer them thoroughly and patiently, and be prepared to address emotional reactions with understanding. The emotional response may require time.

Beyond conveying medical information, effective communication includes actively engaging patients in shared decision-making. Explain treatment options clearly, weighing the potential benefits and risks of each, but refrain from imposing your personal opinion or preference. Empower your patient by presenting them with the necessary information so they can be a key part of the decision-making process. This will increase their likelihood to adhere to treatment. This collaborative approach respects patient autonomy and fosters a stronger physician-patient partnership.

Documentation of patient communication is just as vital as the communication itself. Maintain meticulous records of all conversations, documenting the information shared, the patient's understanding, and any decisions made. This documentation serves as legal protection and promotes continuity of care across providers. The process of the discussion, along with the content, matters.

Finally, recognize the limitations of your own communication style. Seek feedback from colleagues, supervisors, or even patients themselves, to identify areas for improvement. Continuous self-reflection and a commitment to lifelong learning are essential for developing and refining your communication skills, enhancing your ability to provide excellent patient care. Always strive to be a better communicator.

6 Chapter 6: Confidentiality & Privacy

Maintaining patient confidentiality is paramount; it forms the bedrock of trust in the doctor-patient relationship. This trust, once broken, is incredibly difficult to repair, potentially damaging both the individual patient and the broader healthcare system. The consequences can range from diminished patient willingness to seek care, leading to delayed diagnosis and treatment, to legal repercussions for the physician. Therefore, safeguarding this confidentiality is not just an ethical imperative, but a practical necessity for effective healthcare delivery.

HIPAA, the Health Insurance Portability and Accountability Act of 1996, provides a robust legal framework for protecting patient health information in the United States. It outlines specific regulations regarding the use, disclosure, and safeguarding of protected health information (PHI). Understanding HIPAA's provisions—from the definition of PHI to the permitted uses and disclosures—is critical for every healthcare professional. Compliance isn't simply a matter of ticking boxes; it represents a commitment to upholding the highest standards of patient privacy. Failure to comply can result in significant fines and legal action. Beyond simple compliance, though, lies the true ethical spirit of HIPAA—the unwavering dedication to protecting a patient's most personal information.

However, HIPAA isn't a monolithic entity; it acknowledges situations demanding exceptions to confidentiality. Mandatory reporting laws, for instance, necessitate disclosure of certain information, such as suspected child abuse or neglect, to protect vulnerable individuals. Similarly, public health concerns, like communicable diseases, may justify the release of specific information to prevent wider outbreaks. These exceptions, though necessary, must be handled with the utmost care and sensitivity. The physician should be guided by ethical principles, ensuring the minimal necessary information is disclosed, only to appropriate authorities, while upholding patient dignity as much as possible. The balancing act between protecting individual privacy and safeguarding public health is a delicate one that requires careful consideration and judicious decision-making.

Beyond mandated reporting, other situations necessitate thoughtful consideration. Court orders, for example, may compel the disclosure of confidential patient information. In such cases, the physician's role is to challenge unwarranted requests and to advocate for their patient's rights, even while complying with legal directives. This often requires careful navigation of legal and ethical complexities. Collaboration with legal counsel is frequently necessary to determine the appropriate course of action. In other situations, a patient's own actions might necessitate a breach of confidentiality – for example, if a patient explicitly threatens harm to themselves or others. This requires a nuanced understanding of both the letter and the spirit of the law, and a careful weighing of the potential risks and benefits of each action.

The digital age presents new challenges to maintaining confidentiality. Electronic health records (EHRs), while offering efficiency improvements, increase vulnerability to data breaches. Healthcare professionals must be vigilant in safeguarding access to these systems, employing robust security measures and adhering to strict protocols to prevent unauthorized access. Furthermore, the proliferation of personal health apps and wearable devices raises further complexities, requiring thoughtful consideration of data security and patient privacy. This means not only adhering to existing guidelines, but also proactively anticipating and addressing emerging challenges in data privacy. The responsibility extends to staying abreast of evolving technological landscapes and adapting protective measures accordingly.

Protecting patient privacy extends beyond the realm of legal compliance. It embodies a commitment to fostering trust, respecting autonomy, and upholding the dignity of each individual. This means more than just adhering to regulations, it requires a proactive approach. This involves open communication with patients about privacy practices, fostering a climate of trust, and ensuring that privacy concerns are actively addressed. Healthcare providers should actively educate their patients about how their information is protected and what measures are in place to prevent breaches. By taking these proactive steps, the physician not only strengthens the patient-physician relationship but also reinforces the foundational commitment to responsible and ethical medical practice. This proactive approach isn't just a matter of procedure; it's about demonstrating genuine respect for the patient's privacy and building a stronger, more trusting relationship. Ultimately, the goal is to ensure patient autonomy and maintain the integrity of the medical profession. The commitment to patient privacy, therefore, isn't merely a legal or regulatory requirement, but an ethical imperative that underpins the entire doctor-patient relationship.

6.1 HIPAA & Beyond

The Health Insurance Portability and Accountability Act of 1996, HIPAA, is a cornerstone of patient privacy in the United States, establishing strict guidelines for the protection of Protected Health Information (PHI). This isn't simply about forms and procedures; it's about upholding the fundamental trust between patient and physician, a trust built on the understanding that deeply personal information will remain confidential. Understanding HIPAA is crucial for every medical professional.

However, HIPAA is only the beginning. While it provides a robust framework, the digital age presents unprecedented challenges, constantly testing the limits of traditional confidentiality. The sheer volume of data generated and transmitted electronically necessitates a proactive approach far beyond simple compliance. It requires a continuous reassessment of security protocols, a commitment to ongoing training, and a vigilance in adopting emerging technologies designed to enhance, not compromise, privacy. Consider the increasing use of telehealth—while convenient, it requires airtight security measures to prevent data breaches.

Beyond the technical aspects, the ethical implications are equally complex. While HIPAA outlines specific regulations, its application often requires nuanced judgment, a deep understanding of medical ethics, and a commitment to patient well-being. For instance, situations involving mandatory reporting of certain conditions, such as communicable diseases, present a delicate balance between respecting patient privacy and protecting public health. Navigating these complexities demands an ethical framework that goes beyond mere adherence to legal mandates.

Consider a scenario where a patient reveals a history of domestic abuse during a routine checkup. HIPAA mandates confidentiality, but ethical considerations may outweigh legal obligations if the patient is in imminent danger. This requires a sensitive judgment call, involving careful consideration of all factors and potentially seeking consultation with colleagues or legal professionals to weigh all obligations. A purely legalistic approach might overlook the potential for severe harm, underscoring the need for a thoughtful and patient-centered response, ensuring both legal and ethical compliance.

Moreover, HIPAA's focus on the United States means the landscape becomes considerably broader when considering international collaboration or patients with international connections. These situations require an understanding of diverse legal and ethical norms, recognizing that privacy standards and expectations can vary significantly across cultures. A truly comprehensive approach necessitates an awareness of global perspectives and a willingness to adapt practices accordingly. The physician needs to navigate these complexities with sensitivity and careful consideration, always prioritizing the patient's well-being.

In addition, we must address the growing concerns regarding data security in the face of ever-evolving cyber threats. Ransomware attacks, data breaches, and phishing scams pose significant risks, not only to the privacy of patient information but also to the reputation and legal standing of healthcare providers. Staying abreast of the latest security technologies, implementing robust safeguards, and fostering a culture of cybersecurity awareness within the healthcare setting are not optional but essential components of responsible practice. This includes educating both staff and patients on the importance of data security and adopting best practices to prevent breaches.

Finally, the ever-increasing use of electronic health records (EHRs) brings its own set of ethical and practical challenges. While EHRs offer many benefits, including improved care coordination and data accessibility, they also amplify the risks of data breaches and unauthorized access. The responsible use of EHRs demands a thorough understanding of system security features, adherence to strict access control protocols, and ongoing training for medical staff. It's crucial to balance the efficiency and benefits of EHRs with the crucial responsibility to safeguard patient data. This requires commitment to continuous learning and adapting to the ever-changing technological landscape. The ultimate goal is to leverage technology's power responsibly, always with patient privacy as the paramount concern. Staying informed and vigilant in this area is critical for the future of healthcare.

6.2 Exceptions to Confidentiality

Maintaining patient confidentiality is paramount in building trust and fostering open communication. However, several situations necessitate breaching this confidentiality, often to protect the patient or others. These exceptions are governed by legal and ethical frameworks, emphasizing the delicate balance between safeguarding privacy and fulfilling other vital responsibilities.

The most prevalent exception involves the mandatory reporting of certain communicable diseases. Public health agencies rely on this information to track outbreaks, implement preventative measures, and protect the wider community. Failing to report such illnesses, such as tuberculosis or measles, can have severe consequences, both for the affected individuals and society as a whole. This responsibility outweighs the individual's right to privacy, prioritizing the collective good.

Similarly, suspected child or elder abuse necessitates the disclosure of confidential information. Physicians have a legal and ethical obligation to report any reasonable suspicion of abuse, neglect, or exploitation to the relevant child protection services or adult protective services. The potential harm to vulnerable populations outweighs the principle of confidentiality. This reporting is a critical step in protecting those who cannot protect themselves, even if it means revealing sensitive information disclosed in a confidential doctor-patient setting. Detailed documentation of observations and suspicions is crucial in such cases, substantiating the report and ensuring appropriate action is taken.

In situations where a patient poses a credible threat of harm to themselves or others, confidentiality can be breached. This includes instances of suicidal ideation with clear plans, homicidal threats, or imminent self-harm. Informing appropriate authorities, such as law enforcement or mental health professionals, might be necessary to prevent tragic outcomes. The assessment of potential harm requires careful consideration, taking into account the patient's specific statements, behaviors, and overall clinical presentation. This is a complex area demanding careful professional judgment and consideration of potential legal ramifications.

Court orders can compel physicians to disclose confidential patient information. Subpoenas or court-ordered releases require adherence to legal processes, ensuring that information is released appropriately and within the constraints of the legal system. Understanding the legal requirements for responding to court orders is crucial, ensuring compliance while respecting the legal process and patient rights to the greatest extent possible within these parameters. It's vital for physicians to understand the legal scope of such disclosures and any limitations.

Finally, instances requiring consultation with other healthcare professionals necessitate sharing limited patient information. This occurs when a patient requires the expertise of other specialists or when consultations are needed for optimal treatment planning. Here, information sharing is justified by the need to provide comprehensive and effective care, prioritizing patient well-being. The extent of disclosure should be limited only to information relevant to the consultation, respecting the patient's confidentiality to the highest degree possible. Transparency with the patient regarding such consultations is always recommended, wherever feasible and appropriate. In all cases, maintaining detailed records of all information released and the rationale for doing so is crucial for both legal and ethical compliance.

Balancing patient autonomy with the need to protect public health and prevent harm requires careful ethical navigation. These exceptions to confidentiality are not to be taken lightly; they demand thorough professional judgment, careful consideration of potential consequences, and scrupulous adherence to legal and ethical guidelines. The ultimate goal remains patient well-being, even when that requires difficult decisions regarding the disclosure of sensitive information. It is the doctor's responsibility to navigate these complexities with skill and sensitivity, constantly striving to maintain both ethical integrity and a high standard of patient care. Transparency with patients, where possible, can often facilitate trust and understanding. Open communication about these legal and ethical constraints is a valuable component of building a strong and positive doctor-patient relationship. This framework is essential for a functioning and ethical medical system that serves both individual and collective needs.

7 Chapter 7: The Future of Ethics

Technological advancements are reshaping healthcare at an unprecedented pace. Genetic engineering, artificial organs, and sophisticated diagnostic tools present incredible opportunities to improve lives, but also raise profound ethical questions. Consider the implications of gene editing—the potential to eradicate inherited diseases is staggering, yet the long-term consequences remain largely unknown. Who decides which genetic traits are "desirable"? How do we prevent the misuse of such powerful technology, ensuring equitable access and avoiding exacerbating existing social inequalities? These are not merely hypothetical questions; they are challenges demanding immediate and thoughtful consideration. The development of artificial intelligence in medical diagnosis, for example, promises faster and potentially more accurate diagnoses but also raises concerns about bias in algorithms, potential job displacement, and the erosion of the doctor-patient relationship if human interaction is minimized. Responsible innovation requires robust ethical frameworks and ongoing dialogue between scientists, ethicists, policymakers, and the public.
Global healthcare disparities represent another significant ethical challenge. Access to quality healthcare remains drastically uneven worldwide, with significant discrepancies based on geography, socioeconomic status, and other factors. This inequality is not just a matter of fairness; it is a public health crisis. Diseases spread across borders regardless of national boundaries, and neglecting the health of populations in less developed countries ultimately jeopardizes global health security.

Finding ethical and effective solutions requires a collaborative, international approach, recognizing the shared responsibility to ensure equitable access to healthcare for all. This involves addressing issues like resource allocation on a global scale, promoting international cooperation in research and development, and fostering capacity building in resource-limited settings. Innovative financing mechanisms, global health partnerships, and equitable distribution of resources are key aspects of a fairer and more just future of healthcare.

Maintaining professional integrity in the face of increasing pressures is paramount. The medical profession operates within a complex web of regulations, financial incentives, and societal expectations. Maintaining the highest ethical standards requires a commitment to patient-centered care above all else, even when faced with challenging circumstances. This includes resisting undue influence from pharmaceutical companies, prioritizing patient autonomy, and advocating for policies that promote both patient well-being and the integrity of the profession. The temptation to compromise ethical principles for personal gain or professional advancement is a constant threat. Strengthening professional codes of ethics, providing robust mechanisms for reporting unethical conduct, and fostering a culture of ethical accountability are all crucial steps in maintaining the moral compass of the medical field. Furthermore, continuous professional development, including ethical reflection and education, is vital in equipping healthcare professionals to navigate the complexities of modern practice.

Emerging challenges are constantly evolving, demanding adaptability and foresight. The rise of big data in healthcare, for instance, presents incredible opportunities for research and personalized medicine, but also raises concerns about data privacy and security. How do we balance the benefits of using patient data for research with the imperative to protect individual privacy? Developing robust data governance frameworks, ensuring transparency in data collection and usage, and empowering patients to control their data are essential steps in mitigating these risks. Beyond data privacy, we are witnessing a shift in healthcare models, including telehealth and remote monitoring. These innovations offer opportunities to

improve access and efficiency, but they also raise questions about quality of care, access to technology, and the potential for widening existing health disparities. We must ensure that these technologies are implemented responsibly, addressing potential inequities and maximizing their benefit for all. These are just a few of the many challenges that will need to be addressed as we move into the future.
Professional responsibility extends beyond individual actions; it encompasses advocacy for policy changes that promote ethical healthcare. This includes advocating for legislation that protects patient rights, ensures equitable access to resources, and supports professional standards. Healthcare professionals have a unique position to influence policy decisions, bringing their expertise and ethical insights to the table. Engaging in public discourse, participating in policymaking processes, and collaborating with other stakeholders are crucial ways to shape a healthcare system that aligns with ethical principles. This requires not only technical competence but also a strong sense of social responsibility and a commitment to using one's influence to advance the well-being of individuals and society as a whole. This includes advocating for policies that address systemic issues such as health inequalities, promoting access to preventative care, and reducing the burden of chronic disease. The future of ethics in healthcare is not just a theoretical concept; it is a collective responsibility that requires active engagement from every member of the profession.

7.1 Technological Advancements

Genetic engineering presents a profound ethical challenge. The ability to alter the human genome holds immense promise for preventing and treating diseases, but it also raises concerns about unintended consequences and the potential for misuse. Consider the possibility of designing babies with specific traits, a scenario that stirs anxieties about eugenics and social inequalities. The ethical implications extend beyond the individual, impacting future generations and raising questions about the very definition of humanity. Balancing the potential benefits with the risks requires careful consideration and robust ethical frameworks. We must develop guidelines that prioritize safety, prevent discrimination, and ensure that these powerful technologies serve the common good, not just the interests of a select few.

The increasing use of artificial organs and prosthetics also introduces complex ethical considerations. While these advancements can significantly improve quality of life and extend lifespans, questions arise regarding access, affordability, and the potential for exacerbating existing social inequalities. The cost of these life-altering technologies could create a two-tiered healthcare system, where only the wealthy can access cutting-edge treatments. Furthermore, the integration of sophisticated prosthetics raises questions about body image, identity, and the very definition of disability. We need to ensure equitable distribution and address the potential societal impact of these remarkable technologies.

Telemedicine, while expanding access to healthcare, particularly in remote areas, necessitates attention to ethical considerations. Issues of patient privacy, data security, and the quality of remote care must be addressed. Maintaining the same standards of care through digital platforms requires robust infrastructure and effective regulatory frameworks. The lack of physical examination can hinder diagnosis and lead to misinterpretations, while the potential for data breaches poses a significant threat to patient confidentiality. We must prioritize patient safety and ensure that technological advancements complement, not compromise, the quality of care.

Big data analytics in healthcare has enormous potential for improving patient outcomes and optimizing resource allocation. However, the use of patient data requires careful ethical navigation. The risk of data breaches and misuse is significant, necessitating strong privacy protections and transparent data governance practices. Algorithms used to predict patient outcomes or allocate resources must be carefully scrutinized for bias and fairness. This requires interdisciplinary collaborations between clinicians, ethicists, data scientists, and policymakers to ensure responsible use of this powerful tool. Maintaining patient trust requires rigorous safeguards to prevent discrimination and ensure data security.

The proliferation of wearable health technology introduces new ethical considerations. While these devices can empower individuals to monitor their health and make informed choices, they also raise concerns about data privacy, security, and the potential for misuse of personal health information. The constant monitoring of health data could lead to increased anxiety and stress, affecting individual well-being. Furthermore, the integration of such technologies into the workplace or insurance systems raises concerns about discrimination and surveillance. Establishing ethical guidelines that balance individual autonomy with the potential benefits of these technologies is crucial. Transparency and informed consent are paramount in this evolving landscape.

Finally, the rapid evolution of genetic testing raises several ethical questions. The ability to identify predispositions to various diseases presents both opportunities and challenges. The risk of genetic discrimination in employment or insurance poses a serious concern. Furthermore, the psychological impact of receiving potentially life-altering genetic information must be carefully considered. The use of genetic information for reproductive decision-making needs to be approached with sensitivity and respect for individual autonomy. Implementing robust legal protections and providing comprehensive genetic counseling are vital to mitigate potential harms and ensure responsible use of this valuable information. The balance between potential benefits and potential harms requires continuous ethical deliberation and responsible innovation.

7.2 Global Healthcare

Global health disparities represent a profound ethical challenge. Access to essential healthcare services, including vaccinations, sanitation, and treatment for common illnesses, remains dramatically uneven across the world. This inequity is not merely a matter of inconvenience; it's a fundamental violation of the principle of justice, denying individuals in less developed nations the same opportunities for health and well-being afforded to those in wealthier countries. This necessitates a global commitment to equitable resource allocation, transcending national borders and political agendas. The sheer scale of the problem demands innovative solutions and

collaborative efforts among nations, healthcare organizations, and individuals.
Consider the stark reality: millions die each year from preventable diseases, simply because they lack access to basic medical care. This isn't a distant problem; it's a crisis impacting human lives in real time, a persistent, gnawing injustice that demands our attention and action. We must grapple with the difficult questions surrounding how to prioritize resources effectively in a world with finite resources and infinite needs. How do we balance the urgent needs of populations facing immediate crises with the long-term goal of building sustainable healthcare systems?

The responsibility for addressing global health disparities falls upon multiple shoulders. Wealthy nations have a moral obligation to provide support, both financial and technical, to developing countries. This includes investing in infrastructure, training healthcare professionals, and facilitating the transfer of medical knowledge and technology. Furthermore, international organizations play a crucial role in coordinating efforts, advocating for policy changes, and overseeing the equitable distribution of resources. However, these efforts must be guided by ethical considerations, ensuring that aid is delivered in a way that respects the autonomy and cultural context of the recipient communities. The imposing challenge is to craft strategies which are both effective and respectful.

Ethical considerations extend beyond simple resource allocation. The pharmaceutical industry, for instance, faces significant ethical dilemmas. The high cost of life-saving medications often makes them inaccessible in many parts of the world, perpetuating health disparities. This raises questions of pricing practices, patent laws, and the responsibilities of pharmaceutical companies in ensuring equitable access to their products. Should pharmaceutical companies be compelled to provide their medications at reduced prices or even donate them to developing countries? How can we strike a balance between incentivizing innovation and ensuring affordability? These are complicated questions without easy answers.

Furthermore, cultural sensitivity is paramount. Healthcare interventions must be tailored to the specific needs and cultural beliefs of the communities they are intended to serve. Programs that fail to account for cultural differences are unlikely to be successful, and may even cause harm. Understanding and respecting the cultural norms and values of the population you seek to assist is crucial to ethical and effective global healthcare initiatives. Ignoring this factor can undermine the entire process, negating the value of the work.

The pursuit of global health equity requires a multifaceted approach that integrates ethical considerations at every stage. It needs collaborative efforts from governments, international organizations, healthcare professionals, and the global community as a whole. It calls for innovative solutions, responsible resource allocation, and a deep commitment to social justice. Only through collaborative and ethical endeavors can we hope to bridge the gap in global health access and work toward a healthier, more just world. The challenge is immense, but the rewards—a world where everyone has access to essential healthcare—are worth the struggle. It demands a long-term commitment from us all.

7.3 Maintaining Integrity

Maintaining integrity is paramount in medicine; it's the bedrock upon which trust, the cornerstone of the doctor-patient relationship, is built. Without it, the ethical frameworks discussed previously crumble, leaving patients vulnerable and the profession discredited. This isn't merely about avoiding legal repercussions, though that's a significant aspect; it's about upholding the sacred oath you took. It's about consistently acting in accordance with the principles of beneficence, nonmaleficence, autonomy, and justice, even when faced with immense pressure or tempting shortcuts.

The temptation to compromise your integrity can arise from many sources. Financial incentives, pressure from colleagues or administrators, or even the sheer exhaustion of a demanding career can lead to ethical lapses. Perhaps a lucrative research opportunity presents itself, demanding a slight bending of the truth regarding data collection. Maybe a demanding administrator pressures you to discharge a patient sooner than medically advisable due to a hospital bed shortage. Or, you find yourself overwhelmed with your caseload and tempted to cut corners, compromising quality of care. These aren't hypothetical scenarios; these are real challenges facing physicians every day.

Recognizing these potential pitfalls is the first step towards safeguarding your integrity. Regular self-reflection is crucial; it allows you to assess your actions, motivations, and the impact of your decisions on your patients. Maintain a personal ethical framework that you can constantly refer back to; this helps anchor you in moments of uncertainty. This framework should extend beyond simply following the letter of the law; it should guide your actions with principles of empathy, fairness, and commitment to the well-being of others. Ask yourself if your actions align with these principles before you implement them.

Building a strong support network is equally critical. This involves collaborating with experienced colleagues and mentors who can offer guidance during ethical dilemmas, providing valuable external perspectives on challenging situations. Honest conversations and open discussions can prevent ethical blind spots and provide different approaches to patient care that ensure integrity remains at the heart of your decisions. Seeking counsel from ethics committees or professional organizations also offers a resource for navigating complexities beyond the capabilities of your immediate network. Don't hesitate to utilize these resources; doing so demonstrates not a weakness, but rather a commitment to ethical practice.

Furthermore, advocating for ethical change within your institution is vital. If you perceive systemic issues that compromise patient care and challenge your integrity, voice your concerns. This might involve initiating conversations with administrators, engaging in internal policy reviews, or even escalating concerns to regulatory bodies. It's not always easy; it may require courage and persistence. Yet, a quiet acceptance of unethical practices normalizes the behavior and allows the erosion of integrity to continue. Your patients deserve a healthcare system where ethical standards are championed, and you owe it to yourself and your profession to be a proactive force for positive change. Remember, your actions resonate far beyond individual patient encounters; they contribute to the overall ethical climate of the medical field.

Moreover, continuous learning is essential. The field of medicine evolves rapidly, as do the ethical complexities it presents. Staying abreast of the latest research, guidelines, and legal precedents is crucial. Participating in professional development activities, including attending conferences, engaging in continuing medical education, and reviewing ethical case studies, all contribute to a deeper understanding of ethical frameworks and equip you with the tools to make informed, morally sound decisions. This isn't just about professional development; it's about a commitment to constant self-improvement, ensuring that your ethical decision-making remains sharp and responsive to the needs of your patients in a constantly evolving environment.

Finally, remember that maintaining integrity isn't a passive state; it's a continuous practice. It requires conscious effort, self-reflection, and a commitment to upholding the highest ethical standards, even when faced with adversity. It involves actively seeking guidance, engaging in continuous learning, and advocating for change within your professional sphere. By embodying integrity in every facet of your medical practice, you not only protect the welfare of your patients, but also safeguard the integrity of the medical profession itself. The responsibility rests on each individual physician to commit themselves to this ongoing process. Doing so ensures that your work aligns with the principles of compassion, fairness, and patient well-being; fundamental elements for providing ethical and responsible medical care.

7.4 Emerging Challenges

Genetic testing presents a complex ethical landscape. The potential to predict future illnesses, even before symptoms appear, raises significant concerns about patient autonomy and the potential for discrimination. Imagine a scenario where a prospective employer requests genetic information, potentially excluding individuals based on predispositions towards certain diseases. This is a tangible reality, highlighting the urgent need for robust legal protections and ethical guidelines. The potential for misuse extends beyond employment; insurance companies might deny coverage based on genetic predispositions. This raises profound questions about fairness and access to healthcare. We must find ways to prevent genetic information from becoming a tool for discrimination and ensure everyone has equal access to healthcare, regardless of their genetic profile. The debate over who owns and controls genetic data further complicates the issue. Is it the individual, the healthcare provider, or the research institution that holds this valuable information? Establishing clear legal and ethical frameworks for data ownership and usage is vital to preserving individual rights and fostering responsible research.

The increasing prevalence of telehealth presents its own set of unique challenges. While offering increased access to care, especially in remote areas, it also raises significant concerns regarding patient privacy and data security. Maintaining confidentiality becomes more challenging in a digital environment, where data breaches are a real possibility. Ensuring the secure transmission and storage of sensitive patient information requires rigorous cybersecurity measures and stringent adherence to privacy regulations like HIPAA. Beyond cybersecurity, telehealth poses challenges to the doctor-patient relationship. The absence of physical proximity can affect the quality of communication and potentially diminish the empathetic connection crucial for effective care. Doctors must be trained to adapt their communication styles to accommodate the limitations of remote interactions. Balancing the benefits of increased access with the risks associated with privacy and the potential for diminished rapport requires careful consideration.

Artificial reproductive technologies, while offering hope to those struggling with infertility, trigger a complex web of ethical dilemmas. The use of in-vitro fertilization (IVF) and other assisted reproductive techniques raises questions about the moral status of embryos, the potential for genetic manipulation, and the implications for family structure. Consider the ethical debate surrounding preimplantation genetic diagnosis (PGD), which allows for the selection of embryos free from genetic disorders. While offering the possibility of preventing inherited diseases, it also raises questions about the value of human life and the potential for genetic discrimination. Access to these advanced technologies often remains unequal, creating disparities in reproductive healthcare. This disparity raises profound issues of justice and equity, demanding careful consideration of fair access to these life-altering technologies. Furthermore, the societal and psychological impacts of these technologies need thorough investigation.

The rise of big data in healthcare offers unprecedented opportunities for improving patient care, but also brings ethical challenges. The aggregation and analysis of vast amounts of patient data could lead to breakthroughs in disease prevention and treatment. However, using this data requires careful attention to preserving patient privacy and ensuring data security. Data breaches could have devastating consequences, potentially exposing sensitive patient information to unauthorized individuals. The ethical use of big data also requires addressing potential biases embedded within the data itself, which can lead to discriminatory outcomes in healthcare delivery. Establishing robust data governance frameworks that prioritize transparency, accountability, and patient consent is critical to ensuring the responsible use of big data in healthcare. The power of predictive analytics—forecasting disease risk based on patient data—also presents ethical complexities. While predictive models can lead to early interventions, they can also lead to labeling and stigmatization. Balancing the benefits of proactive care with the potential for misuse demands thoughtful and careful ethical reflection.

Finally, the increasing globalization of healthcare presents unique ethical challenges. The movement of patients and healthcare professionals across borders creates complexities in legal and ethical frameworks. Standards of care can vary significantly across countries, leading to ethical dilemmas for providers navigating international healthcare systems. Issues of medical tourism, where patients travel to other countries for cheaper healthcare, also raise questions about access, affordability, and quality of care. These complex issues, global in their scope, demand a unified approach to ethical guidelines and international collaboration to guarantee equitable and high-quality healthcare for all, regardless of location. The ongoing challenge lies in fostering cross-cultural understanding and establishing global ethical standards that respect diverse cultural values while upholding fundamental human rights.

7.5 Professional Responsibility

Maintaining professional integrity is paramount; it's the bedrock upon which patient trust is built and sustained. This isn't merely about adhering to legal guidelines, though compliance is undeniably crucial. It's about consistently demonstrating a commitment to ethical principles in every interaction, every diagnosis, and every treatment decision. This involves continuous self-reflection, a willingness to learn from mistakes, and an unwavering dedication to placing the patient's well-being at the forefront of your actions. Consider your role not just as a healer, but also as a steward of the patient's trust.

The evolving landscape of healthcare presents novel challenges to professional responsibility. Technological advancements, while offering incredible opportunities for improved care, simultaneously introduce ethical complexities. Think about the implications of telehealth, for example, where the traditional doctor-patient interaction shifts significantly. How do you ensure patient privacy in a virtual setting? How do you maintain the same level of personal connection and empathetic care? These aren't trivial questions, rather they demand careful consideration and innovative solutions. Staying abreast of these advancements is not merely recommended; it's a non-negotiable aspect of responsible practice.

Open communication is the cornerstone of maintaining ethical standards. This means fostering a transparent relationship with patients, colleagues, and even regulatory bodies. Don't shy away from acknowledging mistakes, whether your own or those of your team. Transparency builds trust, even in the face of adversity. A candid acknowledgement of a medical error, coupled with a plan for remediation and future prevention, demonstrates a commitment to accountability and patient safety. This proactive approach is far more valuable than attempts at concealment which ultimately undermine patient trust and professional credibility.

Effective delegation of tasks requires attention to professional responsibility. As you progress in your career, you'll likely lead teams and delegate responsibilities. It's essential to ensure that all tasks are delegated appropriately, based on the skills and competence of team members. Overburdening junior staff or assigning tasks beyond their capabilities is ethically irresponsible and could potentially jeopardize patient care. Moreover, you have a responsibility to provide adequate supervision and support to your team members. This includes both constructive feedback and the facilitation of their professional development. A supportive leadership style fosters a positive work environment where ethical principles are consistently upheld.

Continuous professional development is not optional; it's a vital element of upholding ethical standards. The field of medicine is constantly evolving, with new discoveries, treatments, and ethical considerations emerging regularly. Staying current requires ongoing education, participation in professional development activities, and a commitment to lifelong learning. It is the responsibility of every medical professional to engage in this process, not only to improve their knowledge and skills but also to remain equipped to handle the ethical dilemmas inherent in the evolving medical landscape. A responsible professional acknowledges that their learning never ends, making consistent self-improvement a constant practice.

Navigating conflicts of interest is another crucial aspect of professional responsibility. These can arise in many forms, from financial incentives to personal relationships with patients. It's essential to identify and manage these conflicts proactively, ensuring that they don't influence clinical decisions or compromise patient care. Transparent policies and procedures can assist in mitigating these risks. Moreover, seeking guidance from colleagues, ethics committees, or regulatory bodies when faced with particularly challenging situations demonstrates responsible conduct. Prioritizing patient well-being above all else must be your unwavering principle.

Reporting unethical conduct is not just permissible; it is often a necessary component of maintaining ethical standards within the healthcare system. If you witness unethical behavior by a colleague, it is your responsibility to address it appropriately. This might involve an informal conversation, a formal complaint, or reporting to the appropriate authorities. It's important to approach such situations with tact and professionalism, but a failure to act in the face of unethical behavior allows it to continue, jeopardizing patient safety and the integrity of the profession as a whole. Your role extends beyond your own actions; it encompasses the accountability for the whole system.

Finally, advocating for patients' rights and access to healthcare is a core tenet of responsible medical practice. This includes working towards equitable access to resources, championing patient autonomy, and advocating for policy changes that promote patient well-being. This advocacy may involve engagement with professional organizations, policy makers, or community groups. This active participation contributes not only to patient welfare but also strengthens the reputation and integrity of the medical profession itself. The responsible physician isn't just a healer; they are a champion for those who need their care the most.